Safe and Sound

SAFE
and
SOUND

**How Not to Get Lost in the Woods
and How to Survive If You Do**

GORDON SNOW

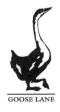

GOOSE LANE

Published by Goose Lane Editions with the assistance of the Canada Council, the Department of Canadian Heritage, and the New Brunswick Department of Municipalities, Culture and Housing, 1997.

The author is grateful for the assistance of his daughter, Nancy MacDougall, and his mother, Irma Snow. Some of the material in *Safe and Sound* appears in slightly different form in the training manuals written by the author for his Search and Rescue courses.

Edited by Laurel Boone.
Cover illustration © Lloyd Fitzgerald, 1996. Reproduced with permission of the artist.
Illustrations by Michael Brislain, 1997.
Author photograph by Geoffrey Gammon.
Cover and interior design by Julie Scriver.
Printed in Canada.
10 9 8 7 6 5 4 3

Canadian Cataloguing in Publication Data
    Snow, Gordon, 1938-
    Safe and sound
    ISBN 0-86492-222-1

1. Wilderness survival.   I. Title.

GV200.5.S66 1997   613.6'9   C97-950061-3

Goose Lane Editions
469 King Street
Fredericton, New Brunswick
CANADA   E3B 1E5

To the memory of George Melvin

CONTENTS

INTRODUCTION

Safe & Sound: How Not to Get Lost in the Woods and How to Survive If You Do is a practical guide to comfort, safety, and survival for all who venture into the woods, whether regularly or only occasionally. The principles have been proven over years of experience by knowledgeable people from all over the world, and the material will acquaint you with how to prepare for your trek and tell you what to do if you should become lost.

In 1956, the Royal Canadian Mounted Police, in the area where I lived, recognized the expertise of my father, my uncle and myself in tracking and searching for lost people. The combined efforts of my family were used on several searches at that time, and I have been looking for people ever since. I joined the RCMP in June of 1957 and retired from that Force in June of 1992. During my service, all within the Province of New Brunswick, I took part in over 200 searches for lost people and actually supervised over 50 such searches. Most of the people that I spent time searching for went into the woods full of confidence, and few were completely ignorant of woodcraft. Yet they all became well and truly lost, lost enough that their loved ones reported them to the local police as being missing, lost enough that it took the RCMP and local volunteers to find them. I now train police, fire fighters, forest rangers and volunteers in search and rescue techniques.

Safe and Sound is intended, not to replace survival training, but to show how to prepare for a trip into the woods so you won't get lost. But everybody who participates in any kind of work or recreation in the woods is likely to get turned around, confused, or even lost once in a while. That's why this book also explains how to stay alive and reasonably comfortable until help arrives. The intention here is to suggest the preparations necessary for a trip into the woods and to outline actions you would need to take to keep you alive until you are rescued.

It's impossible to contain all there is to know about survival in the woods in one small book, and I can't promise that *Safe and Sound* will guarantee that you won't become lost. I hope, though, that it will give you enough self-assurance to survive and indeed care for yourself under all circumstances until you are rescued. If you follow the procedures outlined here, not only will you enhance the chances of your rescuers finding you quickly, but you will also make your stay in the woods a bit more comfortable.

You'll notice that the section on How to Survive is over twice as long as the section on How Not to Get Lost. That's because fixing a mistake always causes more trouble than not making the mistake in the first place.

Safe and Sound is not a complete instructional manual, and it cannot replace field training and experience under competent leadership. Neither author nor publisher assumes responsibility for your safety, and endorsement of specific equipment is based on personal preference only. *Safe and Sound: How Not to Get Lost in the Woods and How to Survive If You Do* will serve as a basic handbook for self-protection. Practise the techniques it teaches.

Not only will they make you a more fully equipped woods person, they will also make life a bit easier for your loved ones who wait at home for your return, safe and sound.

CHAPTER I
HOW NOT TO GET LOST IN THE WOODS

PREPARATION

The best protection against getting lost in the woods is being a good Scout or Guide: Be Prepared. Careful preparation is not only a bulwark against disaster, it's also the best way to enjoy your woods adventures in comfort. Preparation includes knowing what to take with you, what to wear, and how to make sure a search party could look for you effectively. It also includes preparing yourself by learning and rehearsing how to find your way around in the woods. Whether you're hiking, snowmobiling, or berry-picking, your preparations will be much the same.

What to Take

Everybody who expects to spend even the shortest amount of time in the woods should prepare a "ready pack," which can become a survival kit if need be. It doesn't need to contain an elaborate array of expensive equipment but may be prepared from supplies you would normally find in most homes or camps. Take care of your ready pack and carry it with you every time you think you may venture into the woods. If you use any of the contents, replace them immediately upon your return, to make sure your pack is ready for use again.

I always strap on my fanny pack containing the essential items, and you will never find me in the woods without it. In addition to any personal prescribed medication, these essential items are:

- spare knife
- waterproof matches in waterproof container
- Bic lighter(s)
- spare compass
- signal mirror
- flashlight
- whistle
- trail tape & pencil
- space blanket
- plastic garbage and grocery bags
- bite size chocolate chunks
- beef jerky (or similar dried food)

These items take up very little space and weigh practically nothing, yet they can sustain you for several days. A knife is the most useful and important tool you can carry. It can be used for everything from preparing a shelter to whittling a toothpick. A knife will help you bail yourself out of any difficulty, and the spare in your ready pack will protect you against loss, breakage, or forgetfulness. Waterproof matches are priceless. When you really need to light a fire in the rain, ordinary matches just won't do the trick, and paper matches are not much better than no matches at all. Even waterproof matches can become useless if they are carried for any period of time in wet surroundings, so their container too must be waterproof. I also carry a number of Bic lighters. Usually I can get a fire going, even in a downpour, with these devices; however, to be on the safe side, I still always carry my waterproof matches.

Many times, while holding Map and Compass Courses for Search and Rescue people, I have watched participants become so sure their compasses were not working properly that they ignored the readings. I have actually seen an experienced member of the Canadian Armed Forces throw away a perfectly good — and expensive — compass, simply because it was not telling him what he thought it should. Under most circumstances your compass will do what it is supposed to do, but there may be times when you don't believe it. Then you can refer to your second compass. There is always the possibility, too, that you will lose or break your compass, so you should carry a second one anyway, just in case.

A signal mirror is small and compact, and, when used properly, it can reflect sunlight for miles and miles. An aircraft can spot a reflection, even on a cloudy day. You need not acquire a professional signal mirror — any small mirror or piece of polished metal will do. I have seen the lid from a sardine can serve the same purpose as an expensive military signalling mirror. Cut the bottom out of any tin can, punch a hole in the centre, and you have a perfectly good signalling device. You would be amazed at what an effective mirror you can make from a small piece of aluminum foil, even the foil from a pack of cigarettes or chewing gum. All you have to do is press the foil against a small flat surface and hold it up so that the sunlight reflects off it. Then, raising your fingers in the shape of a "V" like a gun sight, find the target to which you wish to send a signal, position your fingers so that the target is in the gun sight, and flash the sun's reflection off your signalling mirror back and forth across your fingers.

I always carry a small flashlight, powered by two AAA batteries, on a cord around my neck. It is not necessary to carry a 12-volt power pack, because you shouldn't travel very far at night unless you know where you are going. You won't have to see very much, and your need for light will be confined to your immediate surroundings or for treating injuries. On the same cord around my neck, I carry a police whistle. The piercing sound of these whistles carries much further than most human voices, particularly at night.

I always carry a roll of trail tape, usually hunter's orange, but sometimes in another colour if orange may already have been used in a particular area for some specific purpose. I put this tape to a multitude of non-emergency uses, from tying my lean-to in place to marking a likely spot for hunting or fishing. I carry the pencil to write notes on the tape. As a rescuer, I have learned that people lost in the woods do not always understand signals that are designed by Search and Rescue people, so I write notes on the tape telling them which way to go to safety.

A space blanket comes folded into a nice neat little package, but, when needed, it unfolds into a double-bed-sized blanket. It will reflect body heat inward or the sun's heat outward and perhaps keep you or some other person from perishing. Space blankets are inexpensive and, even without other equipment, this one article could save your life. Nobody should go into the woods without one.

Plastic garbage and grocery bags have numerous purposes. With a plastic bag you can make a shelter, a water container, a nature still (for making water, not booze), or a complete rain suit. You can keep moisture out of your clothes on a rainy day or keep moisture inside your still on a dry, hot day. Plastic bags are not bulky and will prove to be very useful if you find you have to spend any unexpected amount of time in the woods. One other item of a similar material could also come in handy: a condom. In spite of its tiny package, a condom will hold up to a litre of water for storage, although I would not recommend it for transporting water.

You will *want* a small amount of food in your ready pack, but, to tell the truth, you won't *need* it. Hard as this is to believe, you can live for weeks without food as long as you maintain your body's liquid ratio.

With this in mind, take only a very small quantity of foodstuff, as it is highly unlikely that you will spend any great length of time without either being found or finding something to eat. I carry bite-sized chocolate chunks or the little chocolate bars available at Hallowe'en. These items supply a quick source of energy and the sugar the body seems to crave for a sense of well-being. I also carry a few strips of beef jerky or a similar substance because I can chew on that stuff for hours and it makes me feel as if I'm eating. Don't take these items for a snack while you are hiking; your ready pack is your survival kit, so keep these food items for emergency use only. I know, it seems like an emergency if you have been hiking for six or seven hours without food, but if you do eat any of the contents of your pack, be sure you replace those items before putting your pack away. That way you will be certain that your ready pack is indeed always ready.

If you like, you can add some things that will make a long stay in the woods more comfortable:

- a copy of *Safe and Sound*
- hard candy
- dried fruit
- water purification tablets
- instant coffee or tea bags
- instant soup
- dehydrated meats
- sugar cubes or packs
- instant cocoa
- collapsible drinking cup
- fire starter
- flint
- 1 sq m (1 sq yd) aluminum foil
- chewing gum
- light wire
- 8 m (25 ft) rope
- fish hooks, line, flies
- needle and thread
- iodine
- aspirin
- Band-Aids
- space sticks
- candle
- extra ammo (if hunting)
- spare eyeglasses

As you become accustomed to carrying your ready pack, you will also probably adjust the quantity of any particular item according to your own habits and tastes. You may add other things, but keep the pack small and light so you won't regret having to carry it. Get in the habit of taking your ready pack with you every time you even suspect you may be going into the woods. This little pack will give you confidence while you are travelling in the woods, and, should you become lost, you will have everything necessary to survive almost indefinitely.

What to Wear

Clothing

In days gone by, guides and loggers were well aware of the principles of keeping the body warm. They were active individuals, whether at work or at play, and they knew that bulky garments were a handicap. They knew very well that wool, even when wet, retains body warmth far longer than cotton or any other artificial fabric. Times have changed and the modes of dress have changed with them, but the principles that the early woodsmen applied in keeping warm are still valid and manufacturers still take them into account.

One of those principles is the value of nature's own great insulator — air. Wool insulates so well because it traps a lot of air in its fibres. It is pretty much an accepted fact that the amount of dead air insulation is more important than its source. When dressing for the outdoors, even in today's lightweight clothing, you should pay attention to the dead air principle.

Today's lightweight garments have a remarkable ability to withstand penetrating winds, but often they do not effectively allow for evaporation of perspiration, which can amount to one-half litre (16 oz) of water every 12 hours. While walking, our bodies build up warmth, and we perspire almost continuously. When we stop to rest or stop for the night, unless this perspiration has escaped, it will be trapped in our clothing. This trapped moisture can be a serious problem in a survival situation, because it is essential to maintain body warmth by drying out before retiring for the night.

One way to avoid trapping perspiration is to wear wool and to carry with you a lightweight poncho which will give maximum protection from wind and rain while permitting the body to ventilate thoroughly. A hunter's orange vest over your coat will add more weather protection as well as increase your safety.

Other fabrics as well as wool have valuable properties. *Nylon* is strong even when wet and is resistant to alkali, mildew, and insect damage, and it washes and dries easily. On the down side, it has low moisture absorption, but it will absorb and hold perspiration and body oils. *Gor-Tex*, *Entrant*, and *Klimzate* have tiny holes that allow water vapour to pass out yet prevent water drops from entering. These work well when the wearer is perspiring only lightly, when there is significant temperature and relative humidity difference between the two sides of the material, when the surface is not coated with a layer of water, and when the material is kept clean. *Polypropylene* has excellent insulation power, and it transfers moisture from the body to the outside layer of clothing where it is absorbed or evaporates. This fabric is quick drying, easy to care for, and non-allergenic, and it has a high abrasion resistance. *Polyester* is strong, durable, and inexpensive, it is moisture and rot resistant, and it makes ideal insulation for pants and other clothing articles.

Many types of clothing, both inner and outer, are available today. Don't just go out and buy something because you like the style or colour. Ask questions of fellow outdoors enthusiasts, hunters, or Search and Rescue people and get their opinions. Sometimes sporting-goods store clerks can give you useful advice, though it's important to be alert to their self-interest as well as your own. Based on all the information you can gather, buy what you feel is best suited for your activity, the weather, and the terrain you will be travelling over. I have often seen outdoors people spend good money on outer clothing only to have it ripped to shreds after a few hours of woods travel. I have seen people who could not possibly keep warm when they stopped to rest because all of their clothing was soaking wet with perspiration. You want clothing that is light enough for you to work in, yet with enough insulation value to keep you warm when resting. There is a happy medium for you — all you have to do is find it. No two people are the same, but if you find an article of clothing endorsed by several people engaged in activity similar to yours, the chances are pretty good that you will like it too.

One article of clothing is an absolute necessity: a hat. A great deal of body heat is lost through the top of the head, and you can reduce this loss considerably by wearing some form of head covering. This may not appear to be too important to you as you set off on a nice day. However, when retention of body warmth is crucial to your survival, a hat may save your life. As with other clothing, the choice of material is wide and varied, but any type will prevent some loss of body heat, and, even during cooler night temperatures in the summer, this is important.

Footwear

Footwear is just as important as clothing. Your choice will depend a great deal on the type of activity you will be involved in. A good pair of hiking boots will probably be all you will ever need; however, if you are going to do much travelling through bush and wet terrain, you may wish to find something tougher and more moisture resistant. Again, as with clothing, ask around to see what your friends wear while they enjoy your activity and what has proven to be both sturdy and comfortable. I recommend wearing a boot that will support your ankles.

Rubber boots are waterproof, but they leave a lot to be desired in ankle support, and, because they do not permit ventilation, they are seldom comfortable. Leather boots can be waterproofed, and they are warm, but the waterproofing seals them and prevents any ventilation. Heavy moisture build-up can be expected in both leather boots that have been waterproofed and rubber boots, and they must be well dried after use. Felt insoles will help solve the moisture problem as they will draw the moisture away from the feet and socks, but they must be dried completely before they're used again.

Lighter footwear could be a suitable choice if the terrain is gentle and you don't plan to go far. *Sneakers* or *tennis shoes* provide good support and are comfortable, but they are not moisture resistant, and wetness causes a scalding effect on your feet. *Biking boots* are breathable, light, and comfortable, but they provide no support to the ankles.

Regardless of the type of footwear you choose, you should always carry an extra pair of socks, even when travelling only for a day. They will go a long way toward helping tired feet and warming cold ones. Wearing wet socks can create scalding, and walking with this condition is very uncomfortable.

Leaving Tracks

Now you're equipped: your ready pack is in hand, and you have appropriate clothing and footwear. There's one job left: leave tracks at home.

First, leave actual tracks. Take impressions of your boot tread — or perhaps impressions from all the footwear you'd wear into the woods — and leave them at home. Should you happen to become lost, the searchers would have something positive to look for. This is especially good advice if you're taking children with you, or if your children might stray into the woods by themselves.

Here's how to do it. Place a sheet of aluminum foil on a piece of soft material, such as a folded towel or a pile carpet, and then step on it with both feet. Label the foil with the name of the person wearing that footwear and the date the impression was taken.

Then, let somebody know where you are going and what time you expect to return. This is not a major undertaking, but it is vitally important if you don't return and someone has to go out looking for you. You don't want to be the subject of this typical midnight phone call to the police:

"My husband has not come home yet. Would you see if you can find him?"

"Just what was your husband doing, ma'am?"

"He went hunting."

"Where did he go?"

"I don't know."

"What time was he supposed to return?"

"I don't know, but he's usually home by dark."

Where do the police start to look? What priority should they give to the problem? Do the circumstances warrant a full scale search? They have to ask your spouse a lot of embarrassing questions about your personal habits. Then, when they are satisfied that you are legitimately missing, they have to start looking for your vehicle. Providing you have had the forethought to park it in an open spot and haven't hidden it, they will likely find it within the first few hours, but there's no guarantee. You may be in for a long stay in the woods, and, if you are injured, that just may be too long.

Telling somebody where you are going and when you plan to return is not babyish. Although it is a kindness to those who care about you, it is primarily for your own benefit. At least you will have provided a general area where the police can begin their search for your vehicle. There may be times when you enter the woods for only a minute and don't have a chance to tell anybody. (I have seen people become lost when they just stepped into the woods to answer the call of nature and not been able to find the way to return to their car.) Remember the trail tape you should always carry? Write a note on it and tie it to your vehicle's radio antenna so the police will at least have a starting point when they set out to find you.

MAP AND COMPASS

Usually in the woods you can't see very far, yet you must know where you are, where you're going, and how to get there. Therefore, it is important to take along a map and compass every time you go into the woods and to be comfortable in using them.

Maps

I recommend a topographic map, or "topo" as they are referred to by those who use them. You can acquire these from your local forest ranger office, and they will enable you to form a mental picture of the area you will be travelling in.

A topo is simply a schematic drawing that represents an area as seen from the air, and once you understand the principles, you can read the various symbols and markings. These symbols and lines are all defined on the margin of your map, and all you have to do is take a few minutes to learn what each represents. At least learn to tell at a glance the difference between a stream and a road, a hydro line and the map's own grid line.

Contour lines show graduations in elevation, so you know that where these lines are close together the terrain will be steep, whereas far-apart lines show a gentle rise or fall. Elevations are usually given at even intervals

(10 m, 20 m, 30 m, etc.) and are shown on the contour lines, while dots marking spot elevations show the highest points. The legend of your map will tell you just how much change in elevation the contour lines represent.

Other features on a topo map include highway systems, rivers and streams, lakes, communities, and occasionally buildings and other isolated structures.

By finding the features you can see before you on a map, you can pinpoint your own location. These features function like the signs you will see in shopping malls, airports or other large buildings: they say "You are here." With this in mind, you can easily tell how major landmarks lie in relation to your base of operations and which of them you should be able to see on your route to your destination. Learn the scale too — the ratio between the distance between two points on your map and the actual distance on the ground.

By using the scale at the bottom of your map you can measure the distance between your starting point and your destination. Knowing how far you must travel, you can estimate approximately how long you will take to get there. At home, using a tape measure, mark off a distance of 100 metres and count the number of paces you take to cover that distance. If you will be travelling over different types of terrain, I suggest you do this in each of the types of terrain you will be in, if you can. If your estimate needs to be reasonably accurate, you can carry ten small pebbles in your hand and subtract one for every 100 metres you travel, or start with none and pick up one for every hundred metres.

The direction in which you will travel is determined from the map. You can usually assume that north is at the top of the map and south is at the bottom, but you will also see in the margin arrows pointing to both magnetic and true north. The degree of difference between true and magnetic north is called "magnetic declination." This difference is caused by the fact that the magnetic North Pole is not at the same location as the true or geographic North Pole. The magnetic North Pole is located on Bathurst Island in northern Canada, about 2500 km (1560 mi) south of the geographic North Pole.

North of the equator, your compass needle will point to magnetic north. Magnetic north and geographic north are actually in direct alignment at about Thunder Bay, Ontario. As you travel east of Thunder Bay, your compass needle points more and more to the west of true north. As you travel west of Thunder Bay, your compass points more and more to the east of true north.

The magnetic North Pole is not stationary but continuously moves about, causing changes in magnetic declination. This change is very gradual — only a few degrees in a decade — so don't worry that it will occur while you are taking a reading. To determine the exact declination in your area, call your local forest ranger office.

Compass

You will need a compass to go with your map. Trying to use one without the other is like trying to clap your hands by using only one hand. My favourite compass is the Silva Ranger, which is also used by many forest rangers and search and rescue people and by the RCMP. This type of compass contains all the necessary parts to enable you to use it properly together with a map, including a see-through base, a moveable dial, an adjust-

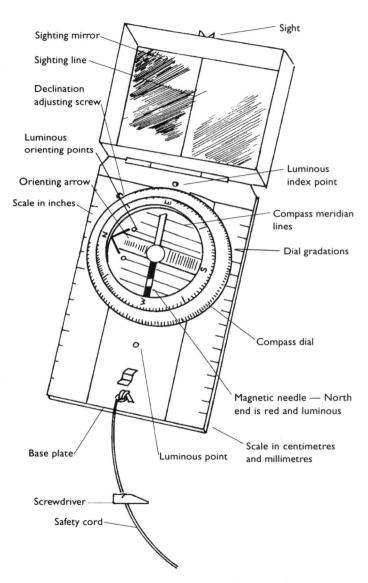

Sighting mirror

Sighting line

Declination adjusting screw

Luminous orienting points

Orienting arrow

Scale in inches

Luminous orienting points

Sight

Luminous index point

Compass meridian lines

Dial gradations

Compass dial

Magnetic needle — North end is red and luminous

Base plate

Luminous point

Screwdriver

Safety cord

Scale in centimetres and millimetres

ment for offsetting the magnetic declination. If your compass lacks this feature, you must always remember that the magnetic North Pole is probably not in the same direction as north on your map. You must calculate that degree of difference and take it into consideration when you determine your direction of travel. If your compass has this offset feature and you have set it properly, you can plan your excursion as if magnetic and true north are the same. This is why I prefer the Silva Ranger and similar compasses, and the following instructions assume that this is what you're using.

First, as soon as you get your map, use a pencil and ruler to extend the true north line all the way up through the map to the top. Then, there are two methods of determining a direction (an azimuth) from a map, and I will describe both of them so you can compare one against the other.

Field Method

This is a field method only. It cannot be done inside a building, over the hood of your car, or anywhere where you will have magnetic interference from areas of metal or hydro lines.

1. Set the magnetic declination on your compass for the area you will be working in. Draw a line on your map between your starting point and your destination.

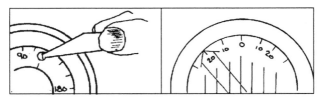

2. Set 360/0 degrees on the hinge end of your compass.

3. Place the edge of the face of your compass along the true north line, *making sure that the mirror end of your compass points toward north.* (Otherwise you will be 180 degrees off and go exactly the wrong way.)

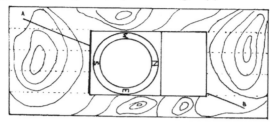

4. Turn the map and compass together until the north end of the needle falls directly into the orienting needle of your compass's dial.

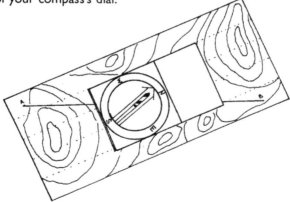

5. Don't move your map. Your map is now oriented, that is, north on the map is the same as true north on the earth. Also, true north now on your compass is true north on the map. The map, the compass, and the earth are now congruent.

6. Place the edge of the face of your compass along your desired line of travel, making sure that the mirror end of your compass points in the direction that you want to travel.

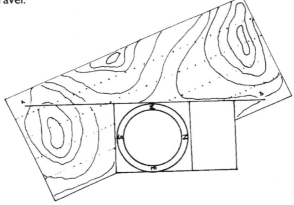

7. Turn the dial of your compass until the north end of the needle falls directly into the orienting arrow of your compass.

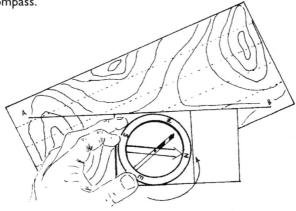

8. Read the dial at the green mark on the hinge end of your compass. This is your reading, the azimuth you will want to use to reach your destination.

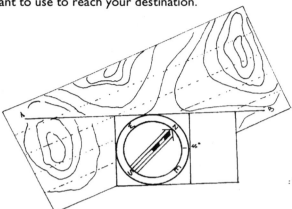

9. *Proceed with caution!* Think your way through! If you think of the four quadrants and know you want to travel in an easterly direction, and you discover you have an azimuth of 270 degrees (that is, due west), you know something is out of whack.

Universal Method

The second method can be used anywhere, and magnetic interference with your compass will not make a difference in your findings.

1. Draw a line on your map between your starting point and your destination.

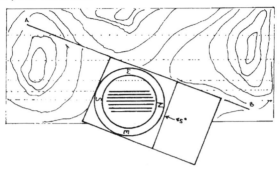

2. There must be a grid line on the map representing true north-south intersecting this line. If not, you can draw in more north-south lines. If you must do this, make sure that all lines you put in are exactly parallel to the original north-south line.

3. Place the edge of the face of your compass along your intended line of travel, making sure that the mirror end of your compass points in the direction you want to travel.

4. Turn the dial of your compass until one of the meridian lines inside the dial of your compass is superimposed on a true north line on your map. *Make sure that north on your compass points to north on your map.*

5. Read the dial at the green mark at the hinge end of your compass. This is your compass reading, the azimuth you must take to reach your destination.

6. *Proceed with caution!* As with the first method, think your way through this before you start travelling.

When you've reached your destination and want to return to your starting point, you'll need a reverse azimuth. To find a reverse azimuth, simply add 180 degrees, but be careful that the total does not exceed 360 degrees. If the total exceeds 360 degrees, subtract 180 degrees from your original azimuth instead. The result will be the reverse azimuth. Don't get in the habit of simply turning your compass around and using the opposite end. This has all kinds of faults, and it is so simple to add 180 degrees to or subtract 180 degrees from your original reading.

If you plan to go hunting in a certain area and intend to use a particular course, you may find all the compass readings at one time and mark them on the map. Later, as you hunt, simply set your compass to the desired headings as you come to each waypoint. This saves time and eliminates errors because you are keeping an accurate log of your trip.

Additionally, when planning a hunting trip, you should mark the boundaries of the area in which you wish to hunt on your map — perhaps a road of some sort on the south, a river on the west, an old railroad bed on the north and a hauling road on the east. This way you won't hunt farther from your starting point than you intended, a wise move if you don't want to spend the night in the woods.

Another good idea for hunters with firearms hunting with a group: decide where each will hunt that day and where he or she will eat lunch. At noon, each fires a shot, with the oldest shooting first. This method accounts for all members of the party at a specific time. You must make contingency plans in the event that someone's shot isn't heard.

Before leaving the road and entering the woods, regardless of your starting point, you should check your compass and heading. You should make certain that the magnetic declination (the orientation needle) has not been moved or damaged. This check shows you which direction the road is running, and, most important, it determines the general direction or course which you must follow to return to the road. (It also assures you that you have not left your compass in your other pants pocket back at camp.) If you follow a deer track for a couple of hours, you can't possibly follow an exact heading back to your starting point. However, if you know that a south-easterly course will put you back on the road, this is all the knowledge you will need to get out of the woods.

Tremendous strides have been made lately in the development of the Global Positioning System (GPS), and I carry a GPS unit whenever I'm in the woods. This little gadget can tell me where I am at any time, and, as well, it can tell me how far I am from my vehicle, what direction it is in, and, at my current speed, how long I will take to get there. You can pre-program a GPS unit to any location without ever having been there, so long as you know the co-ordinates.

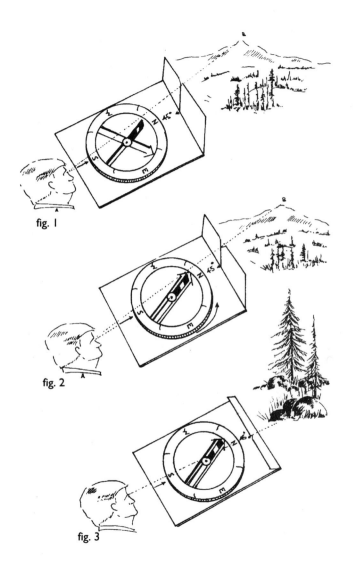

fig. 1

fig. 2

fig. 3

SAFE AND SOUND

Finding Your Way Using Only Your Compass

Many times you will want to walk to a certain spot — a distant hill or some other significant landmark — but you know you will not be able to keep it in sight all the while. There are two ways of doing this: by using the information on your map, or by using your compass.

When you want to find the direction with your compass, face the object or place you will be travelling to, hold the compass in front of you at eye level, and look at the object through the gun sight on your compass dial (fig. 1). Turn the dial of your compass so the north end of the needle is directly over the orienting needle. The reading at the green dot is the azimuth or direction you must travel (fig. 2).

You can now walk from your starting point to your destination even though you go from hill to gully and lose sight of it several times. Pick objects along the way to walk to that are directly in your compass line and walk to one after the other (fig. 3) until you arrive where you want to be. Even if you have travelled this piece of woods before, remember to check every landmark and noteworthy feature against your map. Skip this simple precaution once, and you could be lost for a long time.

The golden rule: *believe your compass.* Unless it is obviously broken, or except under very unusual circumstances, it will do what it is supposed to do.

Improvised Orienteering

Using Your Watch as a Compass

You can use any ordinary watch to help you find the north-south line. This system will work, even on cloudy days.

If the sun is out, point the hour hand of your watch at the sun. A line halfway between the hour hand and 12:00 standard time (1:00 daylight saving time) points south. On a cloudy day, hold a small stick at the centre of your watch so that its shadow falls along the hour hand. A line halfway between the hour hand and 12:00 standard time (1:00 daylight saving time) points north.

A person improvident enough to have entered the woods without a watch or compass, or unlucky enough to have lost them, can still improvise.

Using the Sun as Compass and Watch

In the daytime, you can use the sun to find directions by using a branch or stick to cast a shadow. Find a straight stick about one metre (3 ft) long. On a level, brush-free spot, push the stick into the ground, inclining it to get a longer, bigger shadow if necessary. Mark the tip of the shadow. Wait until the shadow moves a few centimetres (10 to 15 minutes will do). Mark the position of the new shadow tip. Then draw a straight line from the first mark through and about 30 cm (1 ft) past the second mark. Now, put the toe of your left foot at the first marker and the toe of your right foot at the end of the line you just drew. You are now facing true north. Your left foot is at the west end of the line and your right foot is at the east end of the line. South is behind you.

This works because the sun always travels from east to west and so the shadow always moves in the opposite direction.

Another method works on the same principle. Push a one-metre (3-ft) stick into the ground so that it points directly at the sun and casts no shadow on the ground at its base. Wait 10 to 15 minutes; the stick will now cast a shadow. A line drawn between the tip of the shadow and the base of the stick is an east-west line, with the base of the stick at the west end.

You can also use the shadow tip method to approximate the time of day. At the centre of your already-drawn east-west line, draw an intersecting perpendicular north-south line and push a stick into the ground at the intersection. The shadow of the stick becomes the hour hand of your clock and thus you can estimate the time. The stick's shadow would fall on the west part of the line at sunrise (6:00 a.m.) and on the east part at sunset (6:00 p.m.). At noon, the shadow would fall on the north part of the intersecting line. Of course, everywhere except at the equator, while the noon shadow is always true, the other hours will vary somewhat with location and time of year.

Navigating by the Stars

On a clear night, you can use the stars to find directions. To find the North Star, locate the Big Dipper in the northern sky. Visualize a straight line through the two stars forming the outer end of the bowl. Follow along this line about five times the distance between the two stars to find the bright star we know as the North Star.

The constellation Cassiopeia, a group of five bright stars shaped like a lopsided M, or a W when it's low in the sky, can also be used to find the North Star. It is straight out towards the centre of the sky from the middle star in Cassiopeia, at about the same distance as from the Dipper lip. Cassiopeia is almost directly opposite the Dipper; therefore, one constellation or the other will generally be visible so you can find the North Star.

SAFE AND SOUND

CHAPTER 2
HOW TO SURVIVE IF YOU DO GET LOST

A NIGHT IN THE WOODS

No matter how much you prepare, no matter how experienced you are, eventually you're likely to end up not where you thought you'd be. When do you know that you're lost? You may have been feeling uneasy for some time, but you know for sure when you can't deny any longer that night will arrive before you do. Even if you know where you are, but you've been delayed by injuries (or blisters), or you've simply underestimated the time you'd need to get out to wherever you're expected, other people will believe you're lost. Of course, it's possible to realize you're lost at any time of the day, but, since the realization most frequently dawns at dusk, I'll explain how to handle the situation from that perspective.

The first thing to do is to stop, sit down, and gather your thoughts. There's no point in charging through the woods in an unknown direction towards some unknown destiny. Look the situation over and take stock of what is at hand. Decide what should be done first and what can wait until later. Now is the time to prove to yourself that you really are worthy of the title "woodsman."

As you make your preparations to spend a safe and comfortable (if unexpected) night in the woods, keep your ears open even though your eyes will become less and less useful. People may be looking for you. Don't pay too much attention to rifle shots fired at random. If searchers want to get your attention this way, they will fire three well-spaced shots and await a two-shot reply. Be alert for chain saw motors, car horns, a siren, or a whistle — searchers may try to get your attention with any of these, and you, properly equipped as you are, will be able to reply with your own whistle. Answer any sound you feel may be directed to you, but stay where you are. Don't try to walk to searchers; let them come to you. Searchers are likely to have strong lights, but if you try to travel at night you probably will just get in more trouble.

Shelter

Maintaining a constant body core temperature is vital to survival. But you're lost. There are no national park lean-tos in sight. Therefore, you must call upon your ingenuity and improvise a shelter.

Think: what do you need? Your first decision should be the selection of your campsite. In making this choice, you should keep in mind natural shelter. The side of an open hardwood ridge affords little natural shelter from either wind or rain. A better bet would be to find a place with a canopy of green growth on the edge of open hardwoods. Such a site will afford both the shelter of the canopy and an abundance of dead firewood. If the spot you select is near a clearing or shoreline, so much the better, as this open ground would make it easier for you to signal a rescue plane. Also consider the availability of drinking water in picking your campsite, but don't set up near a roaring brook or a waterfall — you won't be able to hear signal shots or your rescuers' shouts.

And don't make camp under a tree loaded with snow, which might come down on you and your fire.

Anything you can use to protect yourself from the elements can be considered shelter. Here is where plastic garbage bags prove their worth. A lean-to can be made by placing poles against a ledge or bluff, and the poles can be thatched with evergreen boughs. This construction, with your plastic bags to waterproof your new home, can make a very comfortable shelter and keep you warm and dry through the foulest weather. You can use dirt and grass to chink holes or cracks and cut down the draft, and you can make a fairly comfortable bed by placing boughs on the ground beneath you.

Your shelter needs to be just big enough for you to get inside without too much cramping. It will take only a few minutes to build, and you don't have to worry about being marked for neatness. A few branches leaned against a low limb and lined with a garbage bag will serve just as well as an elaborate lean-to that would make an entire Scout troop a proud home. Squirming your way in under an old windfall is also a good quick way to find a shelter.

In very hot weather, remember that shade from the sun is your most important daytime requirement. You will need to rest in the shade during the hot part of the day, keeping your clothes on and your head covered. It is also helpful to have moving air — a convection current. Air temperature below the ground surface is up to 40 degrees cooler than the air above ground. A closed metal structure without adequate ventilation, such as a vehicle or storage shed, can become hot enough to kill you. If your stay extends beyond overnight, work during

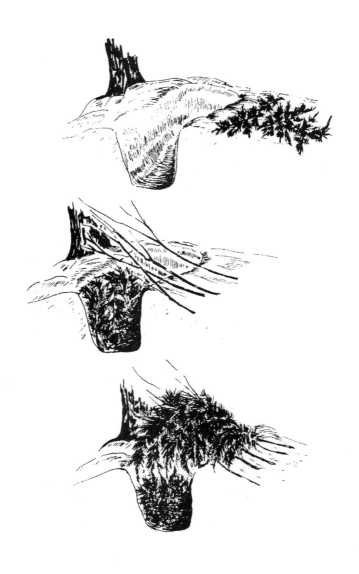

SAFE AND SOUND

cool periods to improve your shelter. Build a fire at night if the temperature drops to an uncomfortable level.

In very cold weather, a fallen tree is the basis of the easiest shelter to construct. It already has a roof, a floor, and one side, and, if there is snow, a shelter may thus be available, already partially made.

In an exposed area, you will have to scrape out a trench in the snow, or, if there is no snow and the ground is not frozen, scrape out a trench in the ground. Pile snow, or rocks or other materials, on the windward side of the trench to make a wind break. Line the trench with evergreen boughs, grass, bark, extra clothes, or any handy insulating material. Cover your trench with snow or evergreen boughs and crawl in. Close the opening if you can to keep your body heat inside.

Snow is a good insulator and gives adequate protection from the wind, but digging a snow cave can take time, and it requires considerable energy. Finding and adapting a snowbank may be less trouble. Either will require work, though, and you must pace yourself to minimize sweating, because you must keep your clothes dry. Ensure that your shelter has ventilation, both to prevent your clothes from becoming damp with perspiration or your breath, and to keep ice from forming. Ice on the inside of your shelter will become a conductor of heat rather than an insulator. I recommend using a candle as a small source of heat, but ventilation is necessary to make sure the candle (or other heat source, if you have one) does not consume all the oxygen.

In extreme cold, shelter should not be taken in ice-coated or metal structures, as metal and ice become conductors and deplete your body heat very rapidly.

Fire

The type and size of your shelter will determine your need for a fire. If you have a small, dry, insulated shelter, you will lose less heat and have less need for a fire. You will have to ask yourself if building and maintaining a fire is worth the cost of the energy it will take.

Rules of thumb:
- The better the shelter, the less need for a fire.
- If your clothing is inadequate, you will require a good shelter.
- If your clothing and shelter are both inadequate, you will require a fire.

You may not absolutely *need* a fire, but you may want one anyway. Most nights get cool enough to make you uncomfortable without a fire, and on a warm evening a fire will make a great signal for searchers. In addition, where man finds work he finds contentment, and gathering firewood is a positive action that will relieve you of the burden of imagined danger.

One in four people cannot start a fire in dry conditions with a match. The reasons for firecraft failure are impatience, inexperience, and poor selection of starter fuels, and the single most important factor in fire starting is the knowledge of fire starters and kindling. Starting a fire in a downpour may seem impossible, but many dried branches, helped by birch bark, a shaved fuzz stick, and some egg carton fuzz balls, will light and burn, even in the heaviest of rain, if given a little shelter.

The Fireplace

The first step in making a fire is to decide where your fire will be. Select an area that is protected from the wind, near potable water, if possible, and near fuel supplies, and prepare your fire spot properly so you won't start a forest fire. Make a fire circle 2 m (6 ft) in diameter on sandy or gravelly soil. A circle of dry rocks can contain the fire, and, if you plan to cook, walling in the fire will concentrate the heat. But never use rocks found in wet areas, such as a stream bed, a swamp, or any other place where they may have been submerged in water. Wet rocks may explode when heat expands any water trapped in their pores. Never build a fire near dry, flammable materials — in very dry grasslands, under overhanging branches, in a very dry forest — or under a snow laden tree, directly on the snow, or on or near wet rocks. A reflector on one side of a fire makes it more efficient, but if you choose a fire site with a large rock surface or at the base of a cliff, do not use the rock as a reflector. Build the fire so that you can sleep between the fire and the rock. The rock will provide warmth on one side and the fire on the other. In colder weather, several small fires built around you heat better than a single larger fire. If a fire must be built in deep snow, build it on a platform of green logs to keep the fire from sinking.

As soon as you decide that a fire is necessary and where it will be, you must gather all your fire material before attempting to start it. Make all your movements count. Even your supply of wood can be used as a windbreak by careful arrangement, and this will conserve fuel as well as reflect heat. You should collect three piles of materials: tinder, kindling, and sustaining fuel.

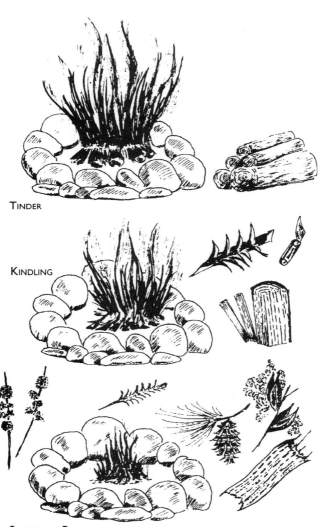

TINDER

KINDLING

SUSTAINING FUEL

Tinder

Tinder is anything that will ignite at a very low temperature with a spark, a small flame or some other heat source. Nature has provided many excellent fire starters. Birch bark is ideal because it contains an oil that will ignite even when wet. Dead tree moss, leaves, and grass also make excellent tinder. When it is raining, your supply of fire starters will prove their worth, and here are some other materials you can use as tinder:

- cotton or scraped cloth
- fine, dry wood shavings
- bird down
- lint or clothing fuzz
- steel wool
- seed down, such as cattail fuzz
- paper
- hair
- dried moss or lichen
- dry, reddish pine needles
- pitch wood, finely shaved or powdered wood
- inner bark of cedar
- candle
- shaved fuzz sticks
- petroleum products or cloth soaked in oil or gas

To make a shaved fuzz stick, select a small dry stick. Begin shaving it from the centre toward the end, but stop the cut just short of the end of the stick so that the shavings are held on.

Use petroleum products cautiously as fire starters. Please be sure you understand their explosive nature and take the necessary precautions.

You can make tinder at home and carry it with you. Try filling the holes in an egg carton with lint from your clothes dryer. Pour melted wax over the lint. You have now created 12 "fuzz balls" that are lightweight, will ignite easily, and will burn for several minutes: excellent fire starters. Other articles soaked in melted wax serve the same purpose: cotton batting, old socks, or almost any cloth. It's smart to carry something of this nature to be used as tinder. So is carrying flint and steel or a metal match as a backup for your waterproof matches and Bic lighter. A common candle is a useful addition to your fire starting kit, as it will ignite easily, it will burn for a long time, and, if you can get it out of the fire, it can be used many times. After you've used your candle to start your fire, you can then use it for illumination.

Kindling

For kindling, find something that will ignite easily from the tinder. It needs to be small in diameter and broken, split, or shaved to increase flammability. Finely split wood, small dry dead branches, or dead dry twigs, which are often available near the base of green trees, are good for kindling, or you can make a fuzz stick. A good supply of kindling should be kept handy in case the fire goes down during the night.

Sustaining Fuel

Sustaining fuel is anything that will burn for an extended period. Generally, it will not ignite from the initial flame, and it requires a high temperature for continued burning. You can use:

- dead wood
- pitch
- dry peat
- coal
- dried dung
- rubber
- green wood
- animal oil or fat
- grass tied into bundles
- petroleum

Be careful of what you choose, because some man-made products, such as Styrofoam, may emit poisonous gases when burned, and others, such as containers, may explode.

Green wood will burn if finely split. If it's dry, nearly all dead wood will burn, and you can find dry wood in the centre of standing dead trees or damp, dead wood lying on the ground. If you have no cutting tools sufficient for splitting wood, whittle a wedge from a piece of hardwood and drive it into weathering cracks in the end of the wood you want to split.

How much wood is needed to sustain a fire overnight? A good rule of thumb is to gather what you think you will need, stand back and have a good look at it, make a guess as to how much wood you have, and then double it, because that's how much you will need. A good test is to measure your fire's consumption for one hour, then multiply that by the number of hours you expect to be in darkness.

Ignition

Now you can build your fire. Arrange the material so that when the tinder ignites, the heat and flame will rise through the maximum amount of kindling. A tepee shape works well. Stack your kindling on end, in the shape of a small tepee about 30 cm (1 ft) high, with your tinder inside the base of the tepee. Now, ignite the tinder.

There are many possible sources of the spark that will ignite your tinder. Learning the primitive skills required to make a spark using friction takes a lot of time, practice and energy, although they give you a great sense of pride when you have mastered them. But modern inventions such as lighters or matches carried in a waterproof container are considerably more reliable and convenient.

Many sporting goods stores carry different types of spark-producing fire starters, such as flints and steels, metal matches, and magnesium fire starters. You can also use your vehicle battery to make a spark. Or you can intensify the sun's light with a magnifying glass, any camera or binocular lens, or a flashlight reflector to start a fire safely.

As your tinder starts to burn the kindling, add larger pieces of fuel. Always start with small pieces and work up to larger materials. Make sure you don't smother the fire by adding too much fuel and cutting off the draft and the oxygen necessary for combustion. As the fire becomes larger and hotter, you can start to put on damper and greener wood.

If you have gasoline or oil available, and also a can, fill the can partially full (about 5-7 cm or 2-3 in) with dry dirt or sand. Then saturate the dirt with oil or gasoline, add a cloth wick, and you have improvised an emergency stove.

Goodnight — Sleep Tight

Even though you're lost in the woods, you've provided yourself with a cosy shelter and a fire. Now for a good night's sleep. To keep nice and warm, you should keep your head covered to prevent the escape of body heat. You should never enter your sleeping area to sleep while you are sweating — let yourself dry off first. You can open your shirt neck, uncover your head, and take off your jacket to cool down, but don't overdo it and get a chill before you retire. If you're short of bedding, remember, thickness combined with dead air equals warmth. Even totally dead dry grass can be used by stuffing it into your clothing or around your sleeping area. Wrap it around your knees, ankles, elbows, feet and chest to help maintain your natural body heat.

Eating sweets before retiring gives a boost to your metabolism which will keep you warm long enough to allow you to fall asleep. Doing light exercises by flexing your muscles, working them against each other without sweating, will stimulate your natural body heat, and then, as you lie down, you will feel cosy and comfortable.

THE MORNING AFTER

Water
Satisfying your body's need for water is critical to survival, and your minimum requirement of two litres (64 oz) a day doubles in hot weather. Obtaining water may

not always be easy, but you can improvise rain water collectors and catch rain in plastic bags or waterproof clothing. In an emergency, you can wring water out of vegetation, devise stills, or dig catch basins for seepage water. Efforts to find water by searching and digging will consume energy and body liquid content, and thus they will increase your water requirement. Drink plenty of water any time it is available, particularly when you are eating.

Remember that your body can lose up to half a litre (16 oz) of water a day in sweat. Therefore it's important to conserve your body fluids by controlling your sweating, especially in hot weather. Keep your clothes on so perspiration doesn't evaporate so fast and so you don't get sunburned. Wear a hat and a neck cloth. If you have a choice, wear light-coloured clothing to reflect light and heat. Stay in the shade during the day. Ration your sweat, not your water!

Where to Look for Water

Along the coast, you may sometimes find water in dunes above the beach or sometimes in the sand above the water level. If not, you can find water by digging a hole just behind the first sand dune from the shore. A damp area in a depression is a likely place. Dig until the hole begins to fill with muddy water, but don't dig too deep or you may get salty water, which is unfit to drink. Let the impurities and suspended particles settle until the water looks clear. Make the water safe to drink by purification and clarification, explained below.

Mountainous or hilly areas are the easiest geographic environment in which to locate water. Most canyons have streams, springs, or intermittent run-off flows during all or part of the year. Dig a hole in a stream bank approximately 2 m (6 ft) from the stream, allow the water to seep in. Wait for it to settle.

If you don't find a stream nearby, look for large rock formations bearing green moss or lush vegetation and seek water at the base. Small isolated clumps of green vegetation in arid regions are good signs of springs. Water is easier to find in loose sediment than it is in rock. Look for springs along valley floors. Benches or terraces above river valleys may have springs or seepages along their bases, even when the stream is dry, and dry stream beds may have water just below the surface. Dig at the lowest point on the outside of a bend in the bed channel. Signs of damp sand along the bottom of a canyon or the base of a hill also suggest that you might get water by digging a seepage hole.

Animals other than humans need water and congregate at good sources. Watch for animals and birds moving in the early morning or late evening. They are probably moving toward water. When an animal trail forks, the best-travelled branch usually leads to water, because animals converge more and more on the same trail as they near a water source. But if you come upon a pond or slough with few or no animal tracks around it and few plants nearby, the water may have a high mineral content which could cause extreme illness. Do not drink it.

How to Distil Water
As long as you have a plastic bag, you can distil your own water using vegetation or the sun. Some garbage bags are treated with anti-fungal or anti-bacterial chemicals, and these should not be used for making a still.

Clear plastic bags are the most efficient. Water produced in a vegetation still will taste like the plants that are used. Whether or not poisonous plants produce poisoned water is still being debated; therefore, I suggest that you not use poisonous plants. Do not drink water that has been in direct contact with the vegetation or that has dripped off of the underside of the vegetation.

Tree and herbaceous plant roots draw moisture from the ground, but a tree may take it from a water table 15 m (50 ft) or more below the surface, too deep for you to reach by digging. You don't have to. You can let the tree do the pumping for you. Choose a tree with healthy vegetation and leafy branches. Place a plastic bag over as much of a leafy branch as you can. Keep the mouth of the bag at the top, and make sure a corner hangs low to collect condensation.

You can do the same with any leafy shrub, or even cut vegetation. Place a plastic bag like a tent over any vegetation. Support the tent with a padded stick upright under the centre, and be sure you have a trough to collect the condensation around the bottom of your tent. Water drawn from the plant by the sun will evaporate and condense on the plastic. As the condensation cools, it will trickle down the plastic and collect in the trough or channels at the bottom.

SAFE AND SOUND

Don't let the foliage touch the plastic, because it will divert the moisture.

Solar stills work slowly and require hot sunlight and patience. Dig a hole 1m (3 ft) wide and 1m (3 ft) deep in the location where water would stand the longest after a rain. Line the bottom of the hole with any green vegetation. Place a water container in the centre on top of the vegetation. Run a tube through which you could suck water, if you have one, from the container out over the edge of the hole. Lay clear plastic over the hole so that it sags down in the centre above the container, and seal the edges of the plastic with dirt. Place a small rock insulated with cloth or paper in the centre of the plastic, directly over the container.

This still can produce half a litre (16 oz) of water in about three hours. Use the drinking tube and open the still only when necessary, as regaining the operating atmosphere inside once the still has been opened takes a long time. Make several stills, if you have the materials.

Water is critical to your survival, and your life may well depend on your ability to find or create it. This is another reason why your emergency kit should contain plastic bags.

Getting Water in Cold Weather
During the winter or in the Arctic, getting enough water to prevent dehydration is as much a concern as the cold. Streams or lakes may provide access to water. If the sun is shining, you can melt snow on dark plastic, a dark tarp, the metal surface of your vehicle, or any surface that will absorb the sun's heat. Whenever possible, melt ice for water rather than snow. You get more water for volume using less heat and in a shorter time. Do not eat

ice or snow; not only is the expenditure of body heat to melt it too great a sacrifice, but, if you eat ice or snow over long periods, the mucous membranes of your mouth will become swollen and raw.

Making Water Fit to Drink

The water you find or make while you're lost in the woods may not be of the best quality and can cause nausea, vomiting, diarrhea, low fever, vague feelings of discomfort, fatigue and weight loss. You do not need any of these symptoms. Therefore you will need to clarify and/or purify your water.

There are several methods to clarify water, depending on your equipment and the water source. If you're getting water from a seepage hole, simply wait for the bits to sink. You can fill several containers with water and let them stand until the sediment has settled, then pour the clarified water off very carefully.

You can filter water by pouring it through several layers of cloth, or you can improvise a filter by putting layers of sand on the bottom of any container with a small hole in the bottom, adding a layer of charcoal and placing a layer of grass on top. Pour in the water, and, as it filters through the contents of your can, it will come out clear.

Remember, clarification is not purification. Clear water can still be contaminated. The best way to purify water is to boil it vigorously for about 10 minutes. Add one extra minute for each 300 m (1000 ft) of altitude. In addition to boiling, you can also use chemical purifiers. Add 4 drops of tincture of iodine to each litre (32 oz) of clear water, or 8 drops to each litre (32 oz) of cloudy water. Or add 2 drops of bleach per litre (32 oz) of clear water or 4 drops per litre (32 oz) of cloudy water. If you use water purification tablets, follow the instructions on the package.

If you must drink questionable water in an emergency, seek medical attention as soon as possible.

Washing
Personal cleanliness safeguards good health by preventing or minimizing internal and external infection and infestation by parasites. Dirty hands can infect any open abrasion and inoculate you with the bacteria in the dirt, and this can lead to infected open cuts or blisters or even to tetanus.

Wash your feet only after the day's work is done, and do not rinse your feet off at travel breaks. I encourage you to take water out of the stream to wash your feet, rather than washing them in the stream. Dispose of wash-water in a cat-hole; don't pour it back directly into the stream.

Signalling

Properly used signals will make others aware of your plight, and the sooner you start signalling, the sooner you will get someone's attention. You must accomplish your signalling without further endangering yourself and in such a way as to improve your chances of being rescued. Your location and distress must be recognized before anyone can rescue you.

The internationally accepted distress sign is a series of three repetitions of any signal — three shots, three fires in a triangle, three whistle blasts — and the response or acknowledgement by the rescuers is two repetitions of any signal.

You can make signals using many different things, and your emergency kit will equip you with some of the materials:

- fire and smoke, natural or canned
- lights
- shadows
- movement
- flags or coloured signalling panels
- dyes
- flares or rockets
- mirrors
- whistles

For maximum efficiency, place signal fires in open areas. Effective smoke signals need to contrast with the surrounding environment: dark against snow, white against dark turf, etc. For black smoke, add to your fire engine oil or rags soaked in oil, plastic, pitch, pitch wood, or pieces of any rubber product. For white smoke, add to your fire green leaves or boughs, moss, ferns, a little water, or wet cloth.

Create an evergreen torch by cutting a small ever-green tree with dense foliage and moving it to the centre of any clearing. Stand it upright and place dry tinder in the lower branches. When an aircraft approaches, light the tree. Smoke, in most circumstances, will shoot up-wards 40 m to 55 m (130 ft to 180 ft).

You can send mirror signals with the purchased or improvised mirror in your ready pack, or you can make any shiny metal, grease-coated unpolished metal, or food tin function as a mirror. This type of signal can be seen for miles even on hazy days.

Shadow signals, for best results, should be arranged in a north and south line and made in an international distress pattern of three, using straight lines and right an-gles.

If you use colour signals, remember that searchers can best see bright colours contrasting with an opposite-coloured background. Bright royal blue contrasts with all environments. Small signal panels or flags are more visible when moved slowly or waved.

Repeated sounds coming from unusual places or at odd times attract attention, and anything audible can carry a vital message that someone is in trouble. Change in landscape, such as brush cut in conspicuous patterns, large lettering tramped in the snow, or rocks piled in regular mounds all spell "help" to rescuers. Anything that will disturb the natural look of your environment is attention-grabbing and could be the signal that attracts your rescuers.

First Aid

Safe and Sound is not intended to be a wilderness medicine manual. This section of the book should be understood only as instruction in how to help yourself or your companions in case of common back country injuries until trained rescuers arrive. Anyone who spends much time in the woods should take the courses in first aid that are available in most communities.

Hypothermia (Exposure)

People can suffer from exposure or hypothermia at any temperature below the normal body temperature; it does not have to be freezing. Symptoms of hypothermia will include shivering and feeling cold, which progress to unconsciousness and, if not treated, eventually to death. The treatment is to warm your body as quickly as possible. You can do this in any number of ways — drink hot liquids, warm yourself by a fire, get out of the wind, change wet clothes to dry, exercise mildly — but you must increase the body core temperature. Avoid caffeine and alcohol. Both promote hypothermia because they dilate the blood vessels all over the body.

Hypothermia is easy to prevent: reduce heat loss and increase heat production. Dressing properly is your most useful tool in preventing heat loss, and mild isometric exercise is the best way to increase heat production.

Bleeding

Applying direct pressure to small cuts will stop the bleeding under most circumstances. To do this, simply place a clean pad over the wound and press hard. You can make a pad out of any clean piece of cloth, such as a handkerchief or shirt-tail. If pressure does not stop the bleeding, apply pressure with your finger(s) directly to the artery feeding the area. If the cut is in the lower arm, you will find the spot to apply pressure — the pressure point — on the inside of the arm between the armpit and the elbow. If the injury is to the leg, you can find the pressure point in the groin towards the front, about where your leg joins your torso. The strong pulse will tell you when you have found the right place. Pressure on these points will usually stop any bleeding on the arms, hands, legs or feet.

If bleeding still persists, use a tourniquet. Make a loop from your belt or a strip of cloth (don't use a wire or cord). Make a pad out of a piece of cloth to place between the tourniquet and the skin to act as a pressure pad and to protect against injury to the tissue. Place the belt or cloth strip about 5 cm (2 in) from the injury, between the injury and the heart; wrap it around the limb twice and tie it off with a knot. Place a stick through the knot and twist the loop until the tourniquet is just tight enough to stop the bleeding. Once the tourniquet has stopped the bleeding, leave it alone; don't remove it.

Fractures
If you are not sure if the injury is indeed a fracture, treat it as a fracture anyway. The most important thing is to prevent the broken bone ends and adjacent joints from moving. Splint the limb by using either saplings or small tree branches to immobilize both the joint above and the joint below the injury. Pad the branches and the limb for comfort. Tie the splint in place with a belt, a strap, or cloth strips torn off clothing, but don't cut off the circulation.

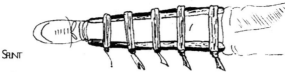

Splint

Sprains

It is common for people travelling through the woods to sprain their ankles. Taping, wrapping, or splinting the ankle firmly over the shoe or boot will permit the injured person to walk short distances without too much difficulty, and you can easily improvise a crutch.

Frostbite

Extremities such as noses, ears, fingers and toes are the body parts most likely to freeze during cold weather. Early frostbite symptoms include slightly flushed skin that later becomes white or greyish-yellow. Either pain or loss of sensation is a warning of impending freezing. Apply warmth, but do not rub the affected part. Warm your fingers or hands in your armpits, then firmly place them over the affected part. Drink warm or hot fluids if they are available. If you absolutely must walk with frostbitten feet or toes, do not thaw them out before you reach medical help. The pain and swelling that accompany thawing might prevent you from putting your footwear on again or even prevent you from walking.

Shock

Shock will often set in after an injury or loss of blood. Symptoms include extreme pallor, cold sweaty skin, severe thirst, and excitability. To help prevent shock, and also to treat it, keep the injured person warm and lying down. Keep the head low unless the injury is to the head, in which case the injured person should recline in a half-sitting position.

Burns

Any burns will likely be minor, but they should not be ignored. Don't try to clean the burn or break the blisters. Unless you have a clean dressing, leave the area exposed. Don't use iodine or antiseptic or apply grease, butter, or cotton to burns. But don't let the burned area get any dirtier, and protect it from sunburn, scrapes, and other further injuries.

Heart Attack

Symptoms of a heart attack include a severe gripping pain in the chest; difficulty in breathing; pain spreading to the neck, to one or both arms, and sometimes to the face; loss of control of normal body functions; profuse sweating; a fluttery feeling; and rapid pulse. If you think you are having a heart attack, lie down with your head slightly raised. Loosen any restrictive clothing to ventilate your body and enable you to breathe freely.

What you do next will be governed by the amount of residual pain after the initial attack passes. If you begin to feel cool, refasten your clothes to stay warm. If you fire signal shots, do not take the shock of recoil on your shoulder — rest the butt of the rifle on the ground. Build a small fire if you're cold and if wood is handy and can be gathered with an absolute minimum of exertion. Even if you begin feeling better, do not exert yourself in any way. Plan your moves carefully. Don't panic. Rescuers will find you.

Woods Travel

When you're lost, you really should stay put to enable searchers to find you quickly. If you have a stalled vehicle, it's likely to be highly visible, and you should stay with it. But, if you absolutely must move on, follow this plan. Leave a note at your campsite. If you forgot your trail tape and pencil, carve a message in a tree or stamp it out in the snow. Then set up sticks or stones pointing in your direction of travel, and mark your trail as you go.

In most areas, there will be an abundance of logging roads, some new and some barely visible, but you will have difficulty in telling which way to go towards civilization and which way would lead you further into the woods. Usually you can determine which way leads to safety by remembering that bulldozers pushed their way in towards the deep woods; trees pushed over on the roadside will lean in that direction. You merely have to walk in the direction opposite to the lean, or against the tree tops. Also, where side roads join the main logging road, the turns will be in the direction of civilization.

You can also follow a brook or stream downstream. The smallest trickle of water, deep in the woods, will eventually end up in the ocean. All you have to do is follow it, and sooner or later you will encounter indications of civilization.

Don't let these woods-travel tips encourage you to try to find your own way out. Remember, except in an unusual circumstance, you are far better off to wait where you are. You will be found.

Edibles in the Wilds

Although you are lost, the chances of being found before you actually need food are excellent. Still, eating makes everyone feel better. There are few places you can go in the world where you will be far from some kind of ve-getation — bush, vine, creeper, flower, grass or lichen — which you can eat to nourish yourself. The only skill you need to make use of these plants is to know which is which and where to find them.

Here are two simple rules to govern your use of edible plants.

1. Leave all mushrooms alone. Mushrooms are mostly water and, from a nutritional standpoint, they aren't worth the gamble.

2. To see whether fruits are edible, cut them horizontally. If they have a star-shaped seed compartment, like an apple, they are edible. But if they have a single seed, like a peach, you had better not risk eating them.

Testing New Plants

I have serious reservations about eating unknown plants. A person can survive for several weeks without any food at all as long as he or she has a supply of water, so finding food should not be a priority for someone temporarily lost in the woods. Although there are no animals in the woods that cause you harm if eaten, there are some plants that will cause you considerable discomfort and may even be fatal. Do you want to take the chance?

Do not assume that, because birds, mammals, or insects have eaten a plant, it is edible for humans. If you feel that eating unknown plants is essential to your survival, test them using the following procedure. Only one person should test each plant. **Never take short cuts. Complete the whole test**. If in any doubt, do **not** eat the plant. Should stomach trouble occur, get relief by drinking plenty of hot water; do not eat again until the pain goes away. If the pain is severe, induce vomiting by tickling the back of your throat. Charcoal from your fire is a useful emetic, and white wood ash mixed to a paste with water will relieve stomach pains.

1. Try to identify the plant.

2. Ensure that it is not slimy or worm-eaten; it will be past its best and have little food value other than the grubs and worms on it, and some plants, when old, change their chemical content and even become toxic.

3. If the plant looks all right, crush a small portion. If it smells of bitter almonds or peaches, **DISCARD.** This is the smell of strychnine, a deadly poison.

4. Rub lightly or squeeze some juice onto a tender part of the body, under the arm between the armpit and elbow, for instance. If you feel any discomfort or see any rash or swelling, **DISCARD.**

5. If the plant does not irritate the skin, proceed in the following stages, going on to the next stage only after waiting at least five minutes to check that there is no unpleasant reaction:

- Place a small portion on the lips.
- Place a small portion on the corner of the mouth.
- Place a small portion on the tip of the tongue.
- Place a small portion under the tongue.
- Chew a small portion, but do not swallow.

If you feel any discomfort whatsoever, such as sore throat, irritation, stinging or burning sensations, itching or swelling, **DISCARD.**

6. Swallow a small amount and **wait five hours.** During this period, eat or drink nothing else.

7. If you have no reaction, such as soreness to the mouth or other discomfort, or digestive problems, you may consider the plant safe. Do not eat large quantities of any one plant at a time, and, if you are not used to eating a plant, start by nibbling a fresh specimen.

All birds and animals are edible, even though some are not too palatable. If you catch either fish or game, you must be sure to cook it thoroughly. If you have a small container for cooking, so much the better. If not, you can fashion a nice cooking pot with your aluminum foil. Cut any meat in small pieces and boil it thoroughly. The broth will have as much nutritional value as the meat itself. If you can't boil it, cut it in small strips and cook it on a stick.

Again, it is important to remember that food is the least of your worries. With plenty of water, your system will sustain itself for long periods with no food or with what you have in your ready pack. Try to keep your mind off your stomach and put your efforts into your shelter or signals.

MIND CONTROL

If you have done everything you were supposed to do, help will be on the way, and all you have to do is wait. In my 40 years of work with Search and Rescue, I've learned that most lost people are found within 12 to 15 hours from the time they are reported missing. Even if you have to stay in the woods for longer than this, there is no need to fear anything out there. You must keep yourself busy and stay in control of your mind and imagination. Fear has a way of working on the mind, and, if you let it, it will create far more evil monsters than have ever actually existed. If you keep your body busy and your mind on what you need to do to survive, everything will turn out just fine. Don't worry too much about food — you now know that you can go for many days without food as long as you have an abundant supply of water. If you have the slightest concern about your safety, don't just sit and worry about it. *Do something*.

You can always gather more firewood or work on improving your shelter. If you are in complete control of your mind, you can just wait, be patient, and enjoy the wonderful peace and quiet of the woods. Help will come, and within a few hours you will be back home with your loved ones telling of your experience.

CHAPTER 3
KIDS IN THE WOODS

Do you take your children into the woods with you? If they enjoy hiking, berry-picking, cross-country skiing, or just plain adventure, they might decide someday to have fun without you. In any situation where you feel that your children might wander into the woods alone, try to take particular note of what they are wearing each day, and be sure to take prints of their footwear.

Of course you should set boundaries for your children and exercise control over their playtime travels and activities. When they're in the woods with you, teach them to stay on a trail, and help them develop an ability to orient themselves by referring to prominent landmarks. Explain the importance of staying warm and dry in all seasons. Encourage older children never to go into the woods alone, but always to go with a partner, and train them to carry a compass and use it. Insist that even teenagers do as you do: tell someone where they're going and when they expect to return. If they change their minds, they should make sure someone knows that, too.

When you take your children on an excursion into the woods, make sure that they, like you, get into the habit of carrying ready packs. At least each child should carry a little food that isn't too tempting and a whistle, which he or she should understand is strictly an emergency signal, not a toy.

TIPS FOR KIDS

Here are a few things you can teach your children to do if they should get lost in the woods.

When you are sure you are lost, remember, "find a space and show your face." Find an open space a clearing where someone has cut wood, a grassy field, or a spot near a pond where no trees are growing.

If people come looking for you, don't be afraid of them. Answer them when they call to you or go to them and tell them who you are. If it is dark, people looking for you make quite a lot of noise. There will be lots of lights and people will be talking. They are your friends, even though they are likely strangers, and they may look funny, especially at night

If a helicopter or plane flies over, look up to it and wave to the pilot. He probably will wave back to you and then fly away to tell the searchers where you are and how to find you. Sometimes it is difficult to see a small person on the ground from a helicopter or airplane. If you are standing in a group of trees, the pilot might not notice you, but in the middle of an open space you will look much bigger. If you lie down in an open field and spread your arms and legs you will look much bigger still. Try to make yourself look as big as you can. If you are wearing bright colours, this will help others see you.

Find a sandy spot or an area with loose dirt and make lots of tracks. You can even write your name. When searchers find this area or a pilot sees it from the air, they will know that you are close by. No one's tracks are the same as yours and your name belongs to you alone. Anybody who finds them will know it was you who made them.

Find a nice tree and stay with it. Your tree should be

near a clearing or open space so you can move into plain sight quickly when you hear a helicopter or airplane coming. Hug and talk to your tree to help keep you from getting lonesome. You must stay in one place.

If a lightning storm comes up, leave your tree and take shelter under lower bushes or blown-down trees. When the lightning stops, go back to your tree.

If it gets dark and you hear noises, yell at the noise and blow your whistle. Bang rocks or sticks together. If the noise-maker is an animal, it will run away, and if it is people looking for you, they will call your name and tell you who they are. Don't try to run away or hide.

Remember that no one is going to be angry with you because you got lost. All your friends will be happy to see you, and your parents will not punish you, so don't hide from the searchers who are looking for you to take you home.

HOW TO HELP YOUR LOST CHILD

It is important to understand that search and rescue teams are highly organized, that a lot of people are going to help you find your lost child, but that you do not have to pay for it. The search and rescue people — the police, forest rangers, wardens, airplane and helicopter pilots, and all the volunteers — are there to help you. They will not quit until your child is found. They will succeed, and much sooner if your child stays in one place and does not panic.

Some children fear or mistrust people in uniform because of the opinions of their families or friends or for many other unjustified reasons. Teach your children that police and other people in uniform are their helpers. Do your best to develop a positive attitude in this regard; it may save their lives if they ever become lost. In this connection, too, you might discuss with your children the difference between the strangers who might harm them and the helpful strangers in a search party.

If your child doesn't return home when expected, or you can't find him or her, call for help immediately. Don't wait. Time lost may mean clues destroyed or the search area contaminated, or bad weather may move in. The distance a lost person travels is directly related to the time he or she spends in the woods, and the closer your child is to your home base the easier the search will be. A call to practically any official organization, such as the forest rangers, Emergency Measures Organization, military, or police will result in the notification of the responsible agency, and they will respond as quickly as they can.

Should your child appear a few minutes later, don't worry that the rescue teams will be upset. They are trained to expect this and would much rather go home knowing that the child is safe with you than spend days trying to find him or her.

Be sure your children know you will do everything in your power to find them if they get lost, and you will not punish them. Teach them that, even if they are lost, they are not abandoned — someone is looking for them. If you know of a successful search and the volunteer effort behind it, or if you read about a search in the newspaper, hear about one on the radio, or see one on TV, tell your children about it. Try to introduce your children to people who are involved in search and rescue. This acquaintance will encourage them should they ever become lost.

CHAPTER 4
SEARCH AND RESCUE

WHAT IS SEARCH AND RESCUE?

If you don't turn up where and when you're expected, the people expecting you — once they've made sure you didn't just sleep in or change your mind — will call the police, and Search and Rescue will go into action.

Search and Rescue consists of locating and aiding persons in distress and relieving their pain and suffering in all its many forms, and the SAR worker has only one aim — to help. Ego building has no place in Search and Rescue. The SAR worker does not expect a bouquet of roses or even feedback from the individuals who benefit from the search efforts.

It's easy to think of search and rescue as a single action, when in reality there are two distinct functions. The search manager is an expert in a sophisticated science involving many modern techniques, including — but not limited to — statistical analysis, probability factors, the psychology of lost people, investigating and interviewing strategies, tracking, and terrain evaluation.

In the rescue component, the search manager focuses on helping a known subject at a known location. Rescuers use a different set of sophisticated technical skills and procedures to remove the lost, stranded, or injured person to safety and, if needed, medical aid.

A Search and Rescue Operation

Search and Rescue workers are trained in the four steps of a Search and Rescue effort: locate the person who needs help; access that person; stabilize his or her condition; and transport him or her to safety. The time involved in any one of the four steps varies with the circumstances.

Locate

None of the other SAR steps can be taken until the missing person is found. Physically looking for the person may be as simple as checking a local address or as complicated as your imagination can dream up. Frequently this function will occupy the greatest percentage of time on any SAR mission.

Access

Once the SAR workers know where the missing person is, they must gain access to him or her. Usually access is simultaneous with finding — the team finds the person when they meet. But this is not always the case. Occasionally the subject is spotted in an almost inaccessible area. He or she may have fallen off a steep cliff along the coastline or became stranded on an island near the coast in heavy seas. Now the major problem, and probably the most time consuming, will be trying to solve the dilemma and actually getting to the subject.

Stabilize

In most cases, stabilization requires only reassurance. This may be easy to administer, but it is very important, particularly if the person requires transportation by litter.

Only properly trained personnel should administer or supervise medical treatment, unless the life of the rescued one depends on it. Stabilization usually takes little time, but, if it involves medical treatment, it may also be very complicated.

Transport

The final step in a SAR effort is getting the subject home, This may be as simple as having him or her follow the searchers back to civilization, or as complicated as evacuating someone off the face of a sheer rock face.

A SAR mission is not complete until all four of these steps have been completed and the missing person has been delivered to safety and is in good care.

The Stages of a Search and Rescue Mission

Every SAR mission will progress through six stages: preplanning, notification, planning/strategy, tactics/operations, demobilization/suspension, and critique.

Preplanning

Good planning means being ready with equipment, an organization framework, and trained workers. All SAR members have an obligation to their organizations to be properly trained, whether they're part of a paid emergency response team such as a police or fire department, or whether they're volunteers. Formal education teaches them what to do under unusual circumstances, but nothing can teach them how to handle the rapid-fire decisions they must make during a quickly escalating mission except the actual experience of being there. Thus preplanning includes pairing inexperienced (though trained) workers with those seasoned in the field.

Notification
Everybody involved in SAR work, no matter how much or how little experience that person has, *must* know how to handle the first report of a situation. The initial actions will certainly affect, and may very well determine, the outcome of that mission.

Planning/Strategy
This component involves the rapid gathering of accurate information so that an assessment can be made of the situation. It applies the basic principles of emergency response and planning to set the tone for the entire search effort.

Tactics/Operations
The tactical component of any SAR mission is the practical application, in the field, of the plans and strategies devised before the search begins.

Suspension/Demobilization
At some point during each mission, a decision must be made to suspend or terminate the mission. Almost every time, this occurs rapidly with the locating and safe return of the missing person. Once in a while, it comes about as a planned activity after days of unsuccessful effort. If the demobilization is planned in advance, the exodus can be organized with little confusion, particularly on larger missions. Most missions that don't meet with quick success are not suspended or terminated, but

are scaled down or continued on a limited basis, sometimes for weeks or even months.

Critique
The information gathered by this means serves as a basis
for revising the preplan and laying a foundation for im-
provement of future searches.

THE SEARCHERS AND RESCUERS

Finding the lost person in the best possible condition is
the prime motivating factor for all SAR operations. This
common purpose serves to draw together a number of
organizations dedicated to serving others as best they
can.

In Canada, whatever police force has local jurisdiction
has the responsibility for conducting any search for people lost in the wilderness. If a person gets lost in a
national park, the park warden has that responsibility.
Ultimately these people, and these people only, must answer for the success (or lack thereof) of any search
within their jurisdiction. They don't work alone, however.
They have a variety of resources that they can call upon
in time of need, depending on what's available in their
area: organizations such as volunteer groups; people
who are expert in tracking other humans; governmental
departments such as the Department of Natural Resources and Energy; search dogs and their handlers;
medical responders; people trained in either water or
snow rescue; people with electronic equipment to help
locate missing persons; the Civil Air Search and Rescue

Association; and pilots who volunteer their aircraft and their time to help in the search.

In New Brunswick, a support plan has been prepared and agreed to by representatives of various organizations which defines what may be expected of each agency. Included in this support plan is the chain of command, should several agencies be called upon at any one time.

Although response may differ around the country, or even within each individual province or state, one factor remains constant: the dedication of the volunteers. In every country, volunteer effort is the backbone to aiding people in distress, and it has proven crucial in wilderness situations. These people, with their skills and their equipment, cannot be replaced by any police agency, or, indeed, any other resource. There are twelve volunteer groups in the province of New Brunswick and anyone interested in joining such a group should call the local RCMP unit for directions to the appropriate person.

Volunteer groups organize their own training workshops. Otherwise very little specific SAR or survival training is available. From time to time individuals offer their services to put on a specific course; however, outside of formal education facilities, such as universities or community colleges, my own company, Search and Rescue Services, is the only source for this type of training in Eastern Canada. In the US there is the National Association for Search and Rescue (NASAR), headquartered in Virginia, and the Emergency Response Institute (ERI) in Olympia, Washington. Instructors from these institutes do travel, and, in fact, Search and Rescue Services has put on several of their courses, upon request, in centres all over Eastern North America. First Aid courses, CPR, and other training necessary for the SAR worker — indeed, beneficial to everybody — can be obtained through the local St John Ambulance Society, Red Cross, or YMCA.

If you love the woods and feel that you'd like to help others who might get into trouble there, call your local RCMP unit to find out how to link up with the Search and Rescue team in your area. If you don't want to be a volunteer — and this kind of work certainly isn't for everyone — please support the team's efforts whenever and wherever you can.

I hope you will never participate in a Search and Rescue mission in the role of the lost person. Prepare yourself properly for the woods so that, if you do get confused, you'll be able to reorient yourself. But never forget — if you do get lost, stay put and follow the guidelines in *Safe and Sound*. The Search and Rescue team will soon be on its way to find you.

THE SEARCH AND RESCUE VOLUNTEERS:
A POEM TO THE PARENTS OF A LOST CHILD

Aw, we've seen it all. We've felt the pain along
with the family when the husband and father
didn't come home,

And we've shared the grief of that young
couple when their child was lost and all
alone.

Our words of comfort are not what you
want to hear us say,

What you really want to hear is that your
loved ones have been found, we're bringing
them home, and that they're okay.

Y'know, organizing a search takes a lot of
time, it just doesn't happen along,

But each little piece of that puzzle has to fit
just right to make sure that nothing goes
wrong.

We don't ask for money or anything else for
what we do,

All we ever ask for or expect is your smile, or
maybe a whispered thank you.

There's not much for you to do when we're
at a search,

So why don't you find a seat and give your
feet a rest?

You just leave everything to us, and you
remember,

We *are the best.*

FOR FURTHER READING

Darman, Peter. *The Survival Handbook.* Toronto: Stoddart, 1996.

Emergency Preparedness Canada. *Self-Help Advice: Prepared for the Woods.* Ottawa: Supply and Services Canada, 1988.

Fry, Allan. *Wilderness Survival Handbook.* Toronto: Macmillan, 1996.

Politano, Colleen. *Lost in the Woods: Child Survival.* Sydney, BC: Porthold, 1984.

Wiseman, John. *The SAS Survival Handbook.* London: HarperCollins, 1986.

FOR MORE INFORMATION ABOUT SEARCH AND RESCUE

Emergency Response Institute
4537 Foxhill Drive NE
Olympia WA
USA 98816

National Association for Search and Rescue
4500 Southgate Place, Suite 100
Chantilly VA
USA 20151

National Search and Rescue Secretariat
4th Floor, Standard Life Building
275 Slater Street
Ottawa ON
Canada K1A 0K2

Search and Rescue Services
763 Glengarry Place
Fredericton NB
Canada E3B 5Z8

PERSONAL RECORD

Please fill in this form. In an emergency, the information could help your rescuers to help you.

Name_____

Address_____

_____

Phone_____

Medical Problems, including medication, allergies and any drug reaction:

_____

_____

_____

In case of accident or serious illness, please notify:

Name_____

Address_____

_____

Phone_____